THE TRANSITION BOOK
I Want to Be Healthy But Where Do I Begin?

Lora A.Reid

THE TRANSITION BOOK
I Want To Be Healthy
But Where Do I Begin?

Lora A. Reid

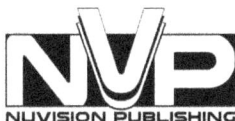

NUVISION PUBLISHING

Books may be ordered through booksellers or by contacting:
Lora A. Reid
P.O. Box 4455
Wilmington NC 28406
www.liftingyourstandards.com

Because of the dynamic nature of the Internet, any web addresses or links
contained in this book may have changed since publication and may no longer
be valid. The views expressed in this work are solely those of the author and do
not necessarily reflect the views of the publisher, and the publisher hereby
disclaims any responsibility for them.

ISBN 978-0-578-19422-6

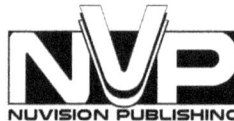

PO Box 4455 | Wilmington NC
www.nuvisiondesigns.biz

Printed in the United States of America.

PREFACE

The information contained in this book is not intended to diagnose, treat, cure or prevent any disease. These statements have not been evaluated by the FDA. In view of the complex, individual nature of health and fitness problems, the information and suggestions in this book are not intended to replace the advice of trained medical professionals. All matters regarding one's health require medical supervision. A physician should be consulted prior to adopting any program or programs described in this book or any of the resources listed in this book. The contents of this book are based on what the author has found to be helpful to her health problems and personal situation. The author and publisher disclaim any liability arising directly or indirectly from the use of this book.

This book is not intended to make recommendations related to getting on or off prescription or over-the-counter medication. If you face any current health concerns, or are currently taking medication, it is always recommended to seek the advice of your physician before starting a new health care program. Only your medical doctor can prescribe drugs or tell you to stop taking your drugs. The role of the author is to make you aware of the hazards of poor lifestyle decisions while helping you to create optimum function and healing in your body. In time, you must begin to judge for yourself whether your medications are keeping you alive, or merely treating the symptoms of the illness not the root cause of the illness. In some instances, the medication may be causing some of the ailments you suffer from. With the guidance of your prescribing physician, you need to make your own best decisions on medication. As you heal, work with your medical doctors to help you reduce or eliminate the drugs you're on.

The information in this book is intended to be educational and should not replace consultation with a competent healthcare professional. This book is intended to be used as an adjunct to responsible health care supervised by a healthcare professional. The author of this book is not liable for any misuse of the material contained in this book.

The products listed in this book are not endorsements. These are products that have helped the author in her healthy lifestyle transition.

Table of Contents

Introduction

INTRODUCTION

This book is about my personal health struggles with experiencing high inflammation, kidney stones, fibroid tumors with menorrhagia and anemia. I was overweight and a pre-diabetic with pre-hypertension. I was able to reverse all of these illnesses by educating myself and transitioning to a healthier lifestyle. It is my hope that I can help others, especially women, who are battling these same problems.

I wish I knew a few years ago, what I know now. Too many of my friends and family have been affected by some type of preventable illness including myself. All of the illnesses mentioned thus far could have been prevented by simple lifestyle changes and being educated about our food and our environment.

There used to be a time when the mention of someone we knew who had cancer was a rarity. Now everyone knows a close friend or family member who has cancer, heart disease or diabetes. These diseases have now reached epidemic proportions in the United States.

If parents can make the necessary changes while their children are young, so many sicknesses can be prevented during their developmental and pubescent years. As adults it will make the pre-menopausal and menopausal symptoms less invasive. My hope and prayer is that everyone I reach can make healthier lifestyle choices for themselves, their children and their parents.

Many people I know say they want to be heathy, but they don't know where to start or what changes to make. Many times, they begin with a New Years' Resolution and go all out but can't sustain their momentum. Other times, they start out by trying to do too much at one time and it becomes overwhelming. For others, like me, we don't attempt to make lifestyle changes until there is a health crisis and we are forced to look at what we are doing to our bodies and pray we haven't done too much damage that would make the health problem irreversible.

I have had some health challenges in the past 10 years which has forced me to make some lifestyle changes. I have found it easier to make small changes first and gradually transition to a permanent life style change.

This book will teach you how to transition into a healthier lifestyle and therefore make it easier to sustain. The items in this book are only what have worked for me thus far, but I am always learning more.

The human body is a self-regulating and a self-healing machine created by God with the necessary systems and processes needed to overcome injury and disease. Nothing will ever be created by man that is more complex than the human body. However, through daily living and exposure to toxic chemicals and environments, our bodies become resistant to self-healing. Therefore, various natural methods of correction is necessary to get our bodies back in line to do what it was created to do.

MY STORY

One day, I was out with a group of friends. Our local church was sponsoring a scavenger hunt for the singles group. It was an extremely hot day in the middle of the summer. I was sweating so hard that the dye from the words on my t-shirt was bleeding down my shirt. I didn't realize how hard I was sweating until someone pointed it out. All of us were sweating but the words on their t-shirts weren't bleeding like mine was. At the time I didn't think much about it because it was so hot that day.

Later that year, I started going to a naturopathic or holistic doctor. One of the items she pointed out in my blood work was how extremely high the inflammation (CRP) marker was for me. The normal range for inflammation is between 1.0 and 3.0 which is the Average Relative Cardiovascular Risk. Mine was well above that at 13.5 which is a sign of infection or chronic inflammation, if it persists. In other words, this signified that my body was very unhealthy.

Mind you, I was seeing a conventional physician at the time and the blood work which he took showed no concerns whatsoever. All of my bloodwork was normal - for what he tested. That is the difference in going to a conventional, western medicine doctor and a naturopathic doctor. The conventional doctor will treat a symptom with synthetic medicine after you develop a disease or health issue. The naturopathic physician will run more thorough lab work and look at pre-cursors that shows what can develop if left unchecked. I would rather prevent the problem with supplements than treat the symptom with medicine. You will never get to the root of the problem when you only treat the symptoms with medication. We need to find out why we have the problem and what can we do to fix it.

The blood work that I received from the Naturopathic doctor showed that I had high inflammation and if I did not change my cating habits, it would develop into diabetes within 10 to 15 years. This didn't develop overnight. It was from years of fried, sugary and salty foods and eating out late at night with friends. I didn't notice the weight I had gained over time. I didn't want diabetes or hypertension or any other health problem. I had to do something to turn this around. Thus, began my healthy lifestyle journey.

To get me started, my doctor gave me a list of foods to eat over a four week period. The first week, I could only eat meat (fish, poultry, beef, and lamb) and vegetables (green leafy). The second week, I could add a few starches (beans) to the list. The third week, I could add some fruit and grains to the list and the fourth week and beyond, I could continue to eat a low glycemic diet. This would help to detox my body and break my bad eating habits which included processed sugars and bad fats.

The first week was very hard but I stuck to it. She also advised me to exercise regularly. This would improve all areas of my health including my inflammation levels. So, I began walking on the nearby college campus a couple of times during the week.

Here's a bit of information on inflammation and why it is so important to get it under control:

Acute inflammation is associated with redness, pain, heat or swelling which occurs in response to things such as joint sprains, ingrown toenails, sore throats or cuts. After that area heals, the inflammation leaves the area. Acute inflammation lasts a short time. However, other issues left uncorrected can force the body into a persistent state of inflammation. With chronic inflammation, the immune system is constantly in distress. A history of inflammation in a particular organ increases cancer risk. For example, cigarette smoke induces a chronic inflammation condition in the lung area which may result into lung cancer.

What contributes to chronic inflammation? Causes of inflammation are linked to excess weight, stress, sleep deprivation, diet and exposure to toxins. Excessive weight increases risk for several types of cancer, including those of the colon, pancreas, liver, endometrium, ovary, kidney, gallbladder and thyroid as well as other types of cancer.

Excessive fat tissue produces high levels of inflammation, which sends a message for the body to repair itself by forming new cells. Rapidly growing cells along with inflammatory secretions damage cells which sets the stage for cancer to develop.

Not smoking and drinking alcohol decreases inflammation. A study in the World Journal of Gastroenterology found that alcohol affects the gastrointestinal tract's ability to keep inflammation-provoking substances out of the bloodstream while also interfering with the liver's ability to detoxify substances created by bacterial infections. Eating a diet that is plant-based, organic and non-GMO reduces your intake of harmful chemicals and helps with controlling your weight thereby decreasing inflammation. Supplements that have proven to decrease chronic information include Vitamin D3 and Curcumin, the substance that gives turmeric its golden-yellow color. By following the diet, she gave me, I was able to slowly lower my inflammation and sugar levels.

One day, I had a terrible pain in my abdomen. The pain was so intense; I had to go to the Emergency Room. By the time the doctor got to me, the pain had subsided. After a few questions about the pain I was experiencing, the doctor told me that their professional opinion is that the pain was probably coming from kidney stones and that they could take a scan, but it would be very expensive. So, I didn't need to get the scan if I didn't want it this time. So, I opted not to get the scan. The pain had subsided.

A few weeks passed and the pain came back. This time, I opted for the x-ray. It showed that my kidneys were full of kidney stones. I was instructed to see a urologist for that problem. The x-ray also showed that I had fibroid tumors in my abdomen as well. I was instructed to see a gynecologist for that problem.

When I saw the urologist, he told me there was nothing that could be done for kidney stones but come back to see him in six months. He gave me a kit that I was supposed to use to strain my urine to try to catch the kidney stones.

By doing this, the urologist could examine the stones and try to determine what caused the stones. I never did catch one.

It was around this time that I had started drinking lemon water, to be healthier, throughout the day. Lemon in water helps the water to taste better. In six months, I went back to the doctor. He looked at my new x-rays and wouldn't say anything. I thought something bad had happened. Finally, I asked him if it had gotten worse. He looked at me in amazement and said, "They're gone". He told me there was only one left and to come back in the next six months. At the next appointment, they had all dissolved.

I thought about what could have contributed to the kidney stones. I realized that it was coming from the antacids with added calcium that I was practically eating every day. Over time the calcium developed into kidney stones. As I changed my diet, I no longer had gas, bloating or indigestion; thereby, eliminating the need for antacids.

I made a visit to the gynecologist to find out more about the fibroid tumors. After having a sonogram, the doctor discussed medical options with me. He told me the tumors were benign and that we would watch them. That usually means we will watch them until they get bigger and then advise you to get a hysterectomy.

All of my friends and family have uterine fibroids or had uterine fibroids at some time in their life between the ages of 25 and 55. Half of them have had surgeries such as a myomectomy to cut them out or a hysterectomy to remove their uterus completely.

What are Uterine Fibroids? Uterine fibroids are tumors that grow in the uterus. The tumors are benign but can cause many problems such as pelvic pain, prolonged menstrual cycles, and infertility. Millions of women experience dysfunctions such as PMS, depression, decreased libido, fibrocystic breasts, food and sugar cravings, irregular or excessive uterine bleeding and endometriosis. Those whose dysfunctions are extremely painful, or debilitating are told that their "health is more important than their reproductive organs" and that "a hysterectomy would be the best thing." Unbelievably, an estimated trillion-plus dollars was spent during the twentieth century to remove women's reproductive organs. Hysterectomy now out-numbers almost all types of surgery performed in the U.S. Uterine fibroids are the leading cause of hysterectomies. In fact, out of every four women in America, three of them usually have fibroids during their lifetime. In the African-American community, 85% to 90% of the women have them. I know this to be true because as I stated earlier, all of my relatives and friends have or had them.

The two symptoms that we all shared are excruciating pain with menorrhagia or excessive bleeding. Those with this problem have menstrual flows that are so heavy that the tampon or pad will need to be changed every hour for at least an entire day, and the cramps are so severe that you are unable to perform your usual activities.

At times, the bleeding was so excessive for me; I would have to go home because I spent all of my time going to the bathroom to change my protection. The pain was so bad; I had to take three Aleve pain pills every 6 hours. I was miserable and anemic.

I worked with my naturopathic doctor to try to find something that would help me. We tried supplements such as progesterone, vitex and maca. The progesterone made it worse and the other two supplements only helped a little, not much.

I tried different remedies that I read on the internet which did help on my heavy days. Taking a tablespoon of Blackstrap Molasses, unsulfured or drinking a couple of tablespoons of apple cider vinegar in water did help slow down the bleeding on heavy days. But these were not long term solutions.

One other practice that I tried that may help shrink fibroids are castor oil packs which should only be applied while not on your menstrual cycle. Castor oil "packs" can be an efficient method of infusing the healing components of castor oil directly into your tissues. I suggest you do a "patch test" prior to applying a castor oil pack to make sure you aren't allergic to the oil.

The process for applying a castor oil pack is as follows. Fold a square piece of flannel so it is still large enough to fit over your entire upper abdomen and liver.

- Soak flannel with the oil so that it is completely saturated. The oil should be at room temperature.

- Lie on your back with your feet elevated (using a pillow under your knees and feet works well), placing flannel pack directly onto your abdomen; cover oiled flannel with a plastic bag, and place a hot water bottle or heating pad on top of the plastic.

- Cover everything with an old towel to insulate the heat. Take caution not to get the oil on whatever you are laying on, as it can stain. If necessary, cover that surface with something to protect it.

- Leave pack on for 45 to 60 minutes.

- When finished, remove the oil from your skin by washing with soap and water. (Be sure to wash the towel by itself, as the castor oil can make other clothes stink if washed together.)

- You can reuse the pack several times, each time adding more oil as needed to keep the pack saturated. Store the pack in a large zip-lock bag or other plastic container in a convenient location, such as next to your bed. Replace the pack after it begins to change color.

- For maximum effectiveness, apply at least four consecutive days per week for one month. Patients who use the pack daily report the most benefits.

This practice helped but until you address the toxins that you are putting in and, on your body, it will not work long term.

The worst. I was now pre-menopausal. I read on the internet that you needed to eat a lot of fiber to flush excessive hormones out of your body. And that to do this, eat a carrot every day and if you eat beef, make sure it is grass fed beef. I started eating a carrot every day. A local restaurant started offering grass fed hamburgers. I thought because it was grass fed, I could eat it without it hurting me. After three weeks of eating carrots and grass fed hamburgers, my next cycle was the worst I had ever had and I lost so much fluid throughout the night, my sister had to call the paramedics to take me to the hospital. They gave me a whole pint of IV saline drip for dehydration in the ambulance before we reached the hospital.

Needless to say, I quit eating carrots and grass fed hamburgers. The carrot is a hybrid vegetable and hamburger is red meat. Neither is good if you have fibroids. At the time, I didn't know this.

I met with my gynecologist to see what else I could do to relieve the problems I was experiencing. He basically said, fibroids were based on heredity and did not offer any solution. In addition, I was 48 years old. The average age for a woman for menopause is 51. During menopause, estrogen levels drop in women and stop feeding the fibroids. They will eventually shrink on their own. I knew that hysterectomies are the number 1 treatment for removing fibroids in America. I was trying my best to hold off a hysterectomy until menopause.

I recently read about Uterine Fibroid Embolizations or UFEs. I asked my gynecologist about getting one. This is a procedure that is gaining much popularity these days. The procedure is similar to a heart catheterization. Patients are asleep during the procedure which takes about an hour to perform.

They receive conscious (intravenous) sedation like you would get during a colonoscopy. Local anesthetic is placed in the right groin/top of the thigh area. A catheter is positioned under x-ray guidance into the blood supply of the uterus. This blood supply can be thought of as a tree with leaves. The trunk is the main uterine artery and the leaves are the branches that supply the fibroids. Tiny particles are injected which are specifically sized for the fibroid vessels. These vessels become blocked, resulting in pruning of the tree. The trunk stays open and supplies the normal uterine tissue, but the fibroids will start to wither away, soften, and eventually shrink in size.

The risks of an UFE are accidental loss of blood supply of surrounding areas causing damage to other organs and it only lasts short term. It may require multiple treatments.

I thought this might work for me. My sister had at myomectomy about ten years ago, but the fibroids eventually came back. I had my doctor schedule an MRI for the UFE procedure, but I was very uneasy about it.

Then I remembered that my sister and a friend of mine had also taken the Lupron shot. It stops the menstrual cycle for three months by decreasing the level of estrogen in the body. Without the blood supply, the fibroids will shrink; at least it did for my sister and friend.

I asked the doctor to cancel the MRI and requested the Lupron shot instead. I thought it would at least give me a break for three months. I took it and the only thing it did for me was give me hot flashes which lasted for seven months after I took the shot. I still bled the whole time.

I kept searching for a solution.

I finally came across some information that finally gave me relief from the symptoms I was dealing with. It was a book entitled, *Got Fibroids, The Fibroid Elimination Bible* by Dr. Amsu Anpu & Dr. Amun Neb. In this book, they explain that estrogen leads to fibroids and many problems that females have including breast cancer and infertility. It also gave information on how to eliminate the estrogen thereby eliminating the fibroids.

My mother was pregnant with my sister and me at the age of 39. While she was carrying us, she suffered with fibroid tumors. Back in the 60's, as today, the answer to fibroids was a hysterectomy. She had one shortly after we were born. At the time, they did not give her hormone replacement therapy which I guess they didn't offer back then. She was fine. She told us she never had any of the symptoms that usually come with menopause such as hot flashes.

Around her mid 70's one of her doctors prescribed estrogen for her to take. She didn't ask any questions and did what the doctor told her to do. A couple of years later, she developed Non-Hodgkin's Lymphoma Cancer which was a side effect of taking estrogen. When she went to the Cancer specialist, they looked at the medication she was taking and threw the estrogen in the trash. She was instructed not to continue to take it. Estrogen has also been linked to breast and ovarian cancer.

She underwent surgery to remove the cancerous lymph nodes under her arm, chemotherapy and radiation. She had to wear a compression sleeve on her right arm for the rest of her life to prevent swelling from the absence of the lymph nodes under her right arm. After she recovered from the treatments, she lived another five years without any problems. The sixth year, the cancer came back. She fought as hard a as she could, but she eventually passed. All of her suffering began with that prescription of estrogen which she did not need.

Estrogen is given to young girls to regulate their periods in the form of birth control pills. The foods we eat and the toxins in our environment promote a build-up of estrogen in our bodies which leads to multiple diseases. Based on the information from several sources, I learned how to decrease estrogen which I will share with you throughout the rest of this book

DETOX

Is your lifestyle toxic?

There are toxins in our environment, air, food, water, cleaning products, cookware and food storage containers. Stress is also a toxin. It's hard for anybody in today's society to not have some stress in their lives. We are surrounded with man-made chemicals with possible cancer-promoting effects according to the public health watchdog Environmental Working Group (ewg.org). Many toxic sources are out of our control but there are some that we can control or at least decrease the amount of toxins we are exposed to.

Before we can promote healing for our bodies, we must first detox and stop putting toxins in our bodies. The primary source of toxins entering our bodies comes through what we consume and what we put on our bodies every day.

How can we stop toxic overload? In this section, we will discuss areas where we can decrease toxins and then what we can do to rebuild our bodies.

Water:

The body is made up of two-thirds water. The benefits of drinking water include weight loss, helps to relieve headaches and backaches due to dehydration, helps in digestion and constipation, less cramps and sprains, and relieves fatigue.

Choose water containers that are naturally Bisphenol A (BPA) free – Glass, stainless steel, etc. Do not drink out of plastic water bottles that contain BPA.

Drink alkaline water which has a pH of 9 to 11 or distilled water. Water filtered with a reverse osmosis filter is slightly acidic, but it's still a far better option than tap water or purified bottled water. Adding pH drops, lemon or lime, or baking soda to your water can also boosts its alkalinity.

Green drinks:

Drinks made from green vegetables and grasses in powder form are loaded with alkaline-forming foods and chlorophyll. Chlorophyll is structurally similar to our own blood and helps alkalize the blood. You can find chlorophyll drops at your local health food store.

Invest in a good water filter for your drinking water to remove chlorine, fluoride and other toxic substances from your tap water. Drinking coconut water is a good choice for hydrating the body, also.

Cookware:

Do not use non-stick Teflon coated cookware which contains Polytetrafluoroetheylene (PTFE). When heated at high temperatures, it releases toxic gases into the air. These fumes are toxic enough to kill pet birds and cause people to develop flu like symptoms (ewg.org).

Use cookware that is Perfluorooctanoic acid (PFOA) and aluminum free. Manufacturers had until the year 2015 to eliminate PFOA from all cooking products. Cast iron, stainless steel and unglazed ceramic are some good replacement options.

Food storage containers:
Do not use soft plastics which contain BPA and Dibutyl Phthalate (DBP). Do not use aluminum wrappings to wrap food unless you first wrap with brown paper or parchment paper. Use non-toxic containers and wrappings – glass, stainless steel, brown paper or parchment paper. Avoid greasy food take out containers or microwave popcorn bags which contain perfluorinated compound (PFCs).

Begin to transition to glass containers for food storage. When purchasing foods in glass jars, wash them out as they become empty and use them to store dried beans, flours, seeds, rice, dried fruit in the pantry or cooked foods in the refrigerator. They can also be used for mixing your home-made creams. They come with their own tops and in various sizes. You would be surprised at the different uses you can find for them when you think about it.

Household cleaners:

Use natural, plant based, non-toxic cleaning supplies. There are many brands out there these days or make it yourself. This is very important for items that come in contact with your skin and in the air you breathe. Avoid Triclosan found in dishwashing liquid, hand soaps and other products listed as anti-bacterial. Check items such as cutting boards, toys and toothbrushes.

Popular Natural Household Cleaning Brands: Seventh Generation, Biokleen, Trader Joe's, Modern, Earth Friendly ECOS, Ambi Powder Cleanser (replaces comet cleanser). An easy DIY multipurpose cleaner can be made by mixing equal parts white vinegar and water. This will clean just as well as store bought products. If the smell of vinegar is too strong, add a few drops of your favorite essential oil.

Stress:

Relieving stress plays a large part in the progress of your healing. Allow your body time to repair. One way to eliminate stress is by being able to say, "No" to things that are not building you up. If we have too much on our plate, we are not getting the proper rest that is required to heal. Our bodies need at least eight hours of sleep. Find ways to release stress and not build stress.

Participate in functions that involve volunteer work. Those who volunteer, have lower anxiety and depression levels. Find a hobby that you can enjoy and that makes you happy. Attend church weekly, pray and meditate.

Eliminate toxic relationships. Make friends with positive people and stay away from negative people. Limit watching the news. Consider individual counseling and group stress management workshops. Find a reason to laugh each day.

Practice deep breathing. Sit outside and eat lunch. Relax by walking in nature, swimming, pursuing creative activities, changing routines.

Oral Hygiene:

Switch to natural toothpastes. You can wet your toothbrush and dip it in baking soda. This will help to brighten your teeth. Or you can mix equal parts coconut oil and baking soda and use as a toothpaste. There are other natural brands of toothpaste available at your local health food store.

Practice regular flossing of your teeth. This is very important for children and adults to clean between the teeth and rid your teeth of debris that the toothbrush may not reach. It will cut down on cavities forming between the teeth.

Get regular dental checkups and cleanings. This protects your gums and teeth from tooth decay and catches any problems early on. If you do not have dental insurance, look for a technical school in your area that offers dental services. Their prices will be much less than other dentists because the dental services will be conducted by students or the dental instructor.

If fillings are required, opt for composite fillings vs silver fillings. Silver fillings are made out of mercury which can lead to poisoning of the system if it begins to deteriorate in your mouth or if accidentally swallowed.

Coconut oil pulling extracts toxins from the body through your mouth. This should be performed first thing in the morning, before brushing your teeth or eating. Take about one teaspoon of coconut oil and place in your mouth. It will melt almost instantly. Swish it in your mouth for about fifteen minutes. When done, spit in the trash. Do not swallow. It is full of toxins. Do not spit it in the sink; it will clog your pipes. If you are battling a chronic illness, do this as often as possible. If you are doing it to stay healthy, you can perform on the weekends.

Coconut pulling will also repair cavities. My sister went to the dentist and she was informed that she was developing a cavity on the gum line of one of her teeth. She would have to come back in a couple of months for them to treat it. I told her to try coconut pulling. She did and when she went back to the Dentist, they could not find the cavity. It works!

Salt Water:

Salt water baths, foot soaks, body scrubs, salt water swimming pools and soaking in beach water. Your skin is the largest organ in your body. By eliminating toxins from your skin, you are detoxing your whole body. Salt naturally extracts toxins. I even heard Martha Stewart say on her show that she soaks her chicken in salt water for two days to draw out the toxins before she makes fried chicken with it.

Massage Therapy:

It does wonders for the body. Technical schools offer discounted massages. In my city, you can get a sixty minute massage for as little as $20. Massage therapy is beneficial for skin, muscles, ligaments, lymphatic system, joints, bones and circulatory, digestive and endocrine system. It helps to relax bodily pressure, nervousness and tiredness. It renews energy. It speeds up blood flow and strengthens the immune system and balances the energy through channels of meridians. It also helps us eliminate waste from our bodies.

Reflexology:

Reflexology is an alternative medicine involving application of pressure to the feet and hands with specific thumb, finger, and hand techniques. It is based on a system of zones and reflex areas that purportedly reflect an image of the body on the feet and hands, with the premise that such work effects a physical change to the body. This is another method of detoxification and promotes healing.

Chiropractic Care:

Your Spine houses the nerves which are connected to each organ in the body. These nerves control everything your body does. It ensures that your body functions correctly. If there is a problem with a certain area of the spine, you may experience problems in certain parts of your body such as tingling or pain. Chiropractors ensure your spine is correctly aligned so that your body can heal itself. Many times, a chiropractor can correct pain in the body without a surgical procedure.

For instance, I had a problem with my right shoulder and arm which is commonly known as frozen shoulder. It was painful for me to lift my arm above my head and quite unbearable. I went to the Chiropractor and in a couple of visits, experienced relief from pain and the ability to lift my arm was restored.

My sister was experiencing tingling and numbness and a feeling of an electrical buzzing sensation in her fingers. She scheduled a chiropractor appointment and after the first visit, all symptoms had ceased.

Choose a chiropractor that will perform a thermal and conventional x-ray. You can see the condition of your spine and the chiropractor can help you reach optimal health. Left uncorrected, spinal issues may result in disease of the area that is not receiving the proper signals from the spine.

Lemon Water:

Drink warm or room temperature water with lemon throughout the day. It will help to detox and dissolve kidney stones if you have any and prevent them from developing. It alkalizes the body, balances blood sugar levels, fights cancer cells and hydrates the lymphatic system. Your liver will love it.

Regular Bowel Movements:

Poop at least once a day, optimum is two to three times a day. Poop is waste. Waste is toxic. Eliminate toxins daily.

Sweat:

It is the body's natural method for detoxification, do not use antiperspirants, only deodorants. A few minutes in a Sauna is good for releasing toxins from the body.

REBUILD

As you detox, you will need to restore and rebuild your body to allow it to heal itself. By allowing toxins in our bodies through food and outside sources, we cause our bodies to stress and overwork our organs. Over time, this promotes sickness and disease. As we begin to implement new lifestyle changes, we can do things to assist our bodies in the healing process and accelerate healing and body repair.

Strengthen Immune System:

A strong immune system helps to fight off diseases including cancer. If you have developed cancer cells, a strong immune system can fight the growth of the cancer cells and prevent them from taking over. Support immune function, thereby reducing stress on the endocrine system.

Drink Noni or Mangosteen juice to strengthen your immune system.

Drink Herbal Tea:

An hour before bed, drink a cup of hot herbal tea with fresh lemon and a teaspoon of raw honey. This prevents colds, flu and sinus infections. Recently, I read that this practice also cuts down on the development of dementia. Choose an herbal tea that will either detox or help you to heal. I drink dandelion tea because it is on the list of foods that are good for an estrogen free diet and can be used to shrink fibroid tumors.

My sister used to be prone to getting sore throats at least twice a year. When we started drinking herbal tea with lemon and honey every night and started taking Vitamin D regularly, she hasn't had a sore throat in several years.

Weight loss and Exercise:

Besides changing my diet, I began an exercise regimen. I purchased an elliptical and worked out on it three to five times a week. I was able to drop twenty pounds in a couple of months. My blood work improved for the better including the inflammation markers which decreased. I was able to drop the weight faster by using the "Interval Method". I like to use the elliptical as my exercise equipment of choice. I use the elliptical for 20 minutes. During the first five minutes, I exercise at a slow to moderate speed to warm up. The next ten minutes I speed up for 30 seconds at a time. Then slow down to a moderate speed for one and half minutes (90 seconds) and repeat until the ten minutes are up. The final five minutes are used to cool down.

In other words:

First 5 minutes – slow to moderate;

Speed up for 30 seconds when your timer hits 7, 9, 11, 13 and 15 and then slow down for 90 seconds;

Last 5 minutes – slow to moderate.

This may be hard to do at first but after a few times, it becomes easier. You will notice the weight dropping off and a loss in inches, especially in the waist and thighs. The Interval Method can be used with walking, biking, or any other exercise method that works for you.

Qigong:

Qigong is a holistic system of coordinated body posture and movement, breathing, and meditation used for health, spirituality, and martial arts training. With roots in Chinese medicine, philosophy, and martial arts, qi gong is traditionally viewed as a practice to cultivate and balance qi, translated as "life energy".

The movements are very simple and easy flowing. This promotes healing from the inside. I was able to find a local meetup group. You may also find short workouts on You Tube or purchase DVDs from amazon.com.

BODY PRODUCTS

Remember -- anything that goes on you goes in you.

I have learned that soy interrupts my hormone balance and I have terrible reactions when I ingest it to include out of cycle, heavy and extended menstrual cycles. I'm sure there are many women who have the same experience but never connected the problem with soy.

I stopped eating foods where soy was one of the ingredients but later realized that I also needed to read the labels of the products I was applying to my skin. They too contained soy. I had tried so hard to control what I ate, only to find out that I was applying it to my skin and absorbing it into my body.

I found soy in my hair oils, Chap Stick, body wash, lotions and other items I probably have not even discovered yet. It's everywhere.

No wonder little girls are developing prematurely; women are having problems with their female reproductive organs in the form of fibroids and heavy bleeding which ultimately leads to fertility problems and hysterectomies. Not to mention disorders that the male population are having but have not made the connection.

Read the labels on your body products and eliminate anything that is harmful to your body.

Ingredients to avoid in Body Products are Soy (Harmone disrupter), Aluminum (found in antiperspirants and is linked to dimentia), Parabens (Xytoestrogen) and Sulfates.

Listed below are personal body products to review and replace as necessary.

Deodorants:
There are usually five toxic ingredients hiding in your deodorant. The first is aluminum which is linked to breast cancer, prostate cancer and increased risk of Alzheimer's

disease. Parabens disrupt our delicate hormonal balance which can lead to things like early puberty in children and increased risk of hormonal cancers. Propylene glycol can cause damage to the central nervous system, liver and heart. Phthalates is linked to a higher risk of birth defects, may disrupt hormone receptors and increases the likelihood of cell mutation. Triclosan is classified as a pesticide by the FDA and classified as a probable carcinogen by the EPA.

A good alternative to your deodorant is to use Crystal Body Deodorant which comes in a stick, roll-on or spray. The only ingredient is mineral salt. It doesn't stop perspiration, but it kills the bacteria that causes odor. Perspiration is a natural process for eliminating toxins from the body. This product is good for both men and women. I found it at my local Whole Foods for about $5. You can also find it on amazon.com.

Toothpaste:
Avoid Fluoride, foaming agents, dyes and chemical

preservatives. Fluoride is toxic which is why most toothpastes carry the warning not to swallow it. If more than a small amount is swallowed, call poison control. Sodium Lauryle Sulfate (SLS) is the foaming agent in toothpaste which can cause a drying effect on the mouth which may increase acidity. It can also cause membrane disruption and trauma in the mouth leading to canker sores. Look for toothpastes without these harmful ingredients.

Adults can practice coconut pulling which can reverse tooth decay. It worked for my sister. For children, have sealants put on the crowns of each tooth. My Dentist applied sealants to my teeth even as an adult. It will prevent cavities from forming on the crowns. Practice good oral hygiene with brushing, flossing and two dental cleanings a year.

Face Toner / Astringent:

Go back to the good old days and use Witch Hazel. For a DIY toner, mix equal parts white vinegar and water.

Face Scrubs:

Read the labels on your face scrub to weed out any toxins that you may be applying to your skin. An easy DIY is to mix equal parts coconut oil and sugar.

Face Moisturizer:

Read the labels on your Face moisturizer to eliminate any toxins. Natural face moisturizers to try are Hempseed or coconut oil which helps fight wrinkles.

Body Wash:

Look for natural body washes or hand soaps made from organic and natural ingredients.

Body Moisturizer:

DIY: Mix 2 cups shea butter, 1 cup mango butter and ¼ cup coconut oil in a blender. Store it in a container.

Body Oils:

You can use avocado, almond or coconut oil. These are especially good during the winter months.

HAIR PRODUCTS

Three years ago, I transitioned from a perm to natural hair. I had no intentions of going natural but decided I was tired of getting perms. I would go to the hair stylist. The stylist would say, tell me when it starts to burn so I can rinse the perm out. I would tell them my scalp was burning and they would say, okay and leave me sitting there for a few more minutes. Why was I paying another person to let me sit in their chair while my scalp is burning?

I decided to stop going to the hair salon and watched a lot of You Tube videos on how to style my hair. I did not want to do the big chop, so I slowly transitioned into natural hair. As my hair grew, I would trim the ends off about a quarter inch at a time until it was all natural.

The problem with going natural is that no two people have the same type of hair. My mother, twin sister and I all had different types of hair. What worked for me, didn't work for my sister. Unfortunately, you have to find what works for your hair.

For me, the flat twists hairstyle worked. This gave the permed hair and natural hair matching waves and made all of my hair look the same until the entire perm was gone.

Ingredients to avoid for Natural hair:
- Soy, Alcohol, sulfates, parabens and silicone.

- Hydrolyzed wheat protein/peptides: Bad for low porosity hair and kinkier Type 4 hair.

- Panthenol/Pro-Vitamin B5: Builds up and acts like protein.

- Glycerin & Propylene glycol: Pulls moisture out of hair cortex in dry conditions, glycerin is also astringent.

- Mineral Oil and waxes: Builds up and is difficult to remove all residues without shampoo.

- Polyquats: Just another version of silicones.

- High amounts of quaternary salts build up.

- Silicones: Builds up, can't be removed without sulphate shampoo.

- Denatured and drying alcohol: Drying to the hair.

- Salts and sulphates: Drying to the hair; sodium hydroxide or any form of lye or hydroxide/ NaOH: Lye, dissolves hair after long term use.

Natural Hair Products to try:

Trader Joes Tea Tree Shampoo/Conditioner

Tresemme Naturals Shampoo/Conditioner

Kinky Curly Knot Today Shampoo/Conditioner

As I Am Shampoo/Conditioner

Camille Rose Naturals Shampoo/Conditioner

Giovanni's L.A. Natural Styling Gel

Kinky Curly Knot Today Curling Custard

As I Am Curling Jelly

Camille Rose Naturals Curl Maker

Design Essentials Curling Custard

My hair was thinning and when I washed it, I noticed more than normal amounts came out when I combed it. I started massaging my scalp with Black Castor oil two to three times a week in the morning before I left for work. After one week, my hair stopped shedding and over time, I noticed my hair started to thicken.

The castor oil has a strong smell, so I put a few drops of peppermint essential oil in it. This improved the smell of the oil. Peppermint oil is also a hair growth stimulant but should be used with a carrier oil such as the castor oil.

FOOD

How important is the food we eat? It's very important. The saying that we are what we eat is true. We can see that in our blood work when we go to the doctor. If we eat foods with a high animal fat content, our cholesterol is high. If we eat a lot of foods with high simple sugar content, our glucose levels are high.

Logically, if we improve what we eat, we can improve our health and, in some cases, reverse the damage that we have done to our bodies. Seventy-five percent of chronic diseases in the United States are related to diet. The biggest culprit is packaged and fast food. The consumption of meat in America is extremely high compared to other modern countries. Americans consume 10 Billion animals and 33 million cows annually.

How can we transition to a better diet? The first step is to learn about the foods you are consuming. Below, list the types of food that everyone should be familiar with to make an informed decision about what they are eating.

Organic, conventionally grown and Genetically Modified Organism (GMO) produce:

When we purchase fruits and vegetables in the produce section of the grocery store, you may or may not have noticed there is a code on each piece of fruit or vegetable. Personally, I had not thought these codes meant anything to the consumer but thought the code was for the scanner at the check-out counter to price the food item. This is true but it also carries another valuable piece of information. It tells the consumer if the food is organic, conventionally grown or a GMO. This information is very important if you wish to transition to a healthier lifestyle. Let's discuss what each type of food means to the consumer.

Organic:

If the code on the label of the food item begins with a 9, the food is organically grown. This means pesticides were not used to grow the fruit or vegetable. This would be the best food to purchase when possible.

Conventional:

If the code on the label of the produce begins with a 4 or 5, the food was grown in the conventional manner with the use of synthetic chemicals and pesticides.

The USDA found a total of 178 different pesticides and pesticide breakdown products on the thousands of produce samples it analyzed. The pesticides persisted on fruits and vegetables even when they were washed and, in some cases, peeled. The EWG's annual Shopper's Guide to Pesticides in Produce™ lists the Dirty Dozen™ fruits and vegetables with the most pesticide residues, and the Clean Fifteen™ where few or no residues were detected.

When buying organic produce is not an option, use the Shopper's Guide to choose foods lower in pesticide residues. With the Shopper's Guide, you can have the health benefits of a diet rich in fruits and vegetables while limiting your exposure to pesticides.

The Dirty Dozen™:

In 2017, EWG's Dirty Dozen list singled out produce with the highest loads of pesticide residues. This year, the list in ranking order includes strawberries, spinach, nectarines, apples, peaches, celery, grapes, pears, cherries, tomatoes, sweet bell peppers and potatoes. A single sample of strawberries showed 20 different pesticides. Spinach samples had, on average, twice as much pesticide residue by weight than any other crop. Pears and potatoes were new additions to the Dirty Dozen, displacing cherry tomatoes and cucumbers from last year's list. These are the top twelve foods where organic or locally grown produce matters.

Dirty Dozen PLUS™:

EWG expanded the Dirty Dozen list to highlight hot peppers, which do not meet their traditional ranking criteria but were found to be contaminated with insecticides toxic to the human nervous system. USDA tests of 739 samples of hot peppers in 2010 and 2011 found residues of three highly toxic insecticides - acephate, chlorpyrifos and oxamyl - on a portion of sampled peppers at concentrations high enough to cause concern. These insecticides are banned on some crops but still allowed on hot peppers. In 2015, California regulators tested 72 unwashed hot peppers and found that residues of these three pesticides are still occasionally detected on the crop. EWG recommends that people who frequently eat hot peppers buy organic. If you cannot find or afford organic hot peppers, cook them, because pesticide levels typically diminish when food is cooked.

The Clean Fifteen™:

EWG's Clean Fifteen list of produce least likely to contain pesticide residues included sweet corn, avocados, pineapples, cabbage, onions, frozen sweet peas, papayas, asparagus, mangoes, eggplant, honeydew melon, kiwis, cantaloupe, cauliflower and grapefruit. Relatively few pesticides were detected on these foods, and tests found low total concentrations of pesticide residues on them. Avocados and sweet corn were the cleanest: only 1 percent of samples showed any detectable pesticides. More than 80 percent of pineapples, papayas, asparagus, onions and cabbage had no pesticide residues. Multiple pesticide residues are extremely rare on Clean Fifteen vegetables. Only 5 percent of Clean Fifteen vegetable samples had two or more pesticides.

How consumers can avoid pesticides:

Smart shopping choices matter. People who eat organic produce eat fewer pesticides. A 2015 study by Cynthia Curl of the University of Washington found that people who report they "often or always" buy organic produce had significantly less organophosphate insecticides in their urine samples. This was true even though they reported eating 70 percent more servings of fruits and vegetables per day than adults reporting they "rarely or never" purchase organic produce. Several long-term observational studies have indicated that organophosphate insecticides may impair children's brain development.

In 2012, the American Academy of Pediatrics issued an important report that said children have "unique susceptibilities to ['pesticide residues'] potential toxicity." The pediatricians' organization cited research that linked pesticide exposures in early life to "pediatric cancers, decreased cognitive function, and behavioral problems." It advised its members to urge parents to consult "reliable resources that provide information on the relative pesticide content of various fruits and vegetables." A key resource it cited was EWG's Shopper's Guide to Pesticides in Produce.

GMO:

Finally, if the code starts with an 8, the food is a GMO or Genetically Modified Organism which means the seeds were genetically engineered or altered by changing their DNA. The pesticides are inside the seeds not on the outside. The first genetically modified plant was introduced in 1982 and since then GMO crops have grown exponentially. They were initially created to withstand extreme conditions of drought and pest infestation. More than 60 countries around the world have banned the sale of GMO foods in their countries.

In contrast, two of the top two GMO products in America can be found in 70% of packaged foods, corn and soy. Other GMO products that are widely used in commercial products are canola, cotton and sugar beets. These items are commonly used as fillers in grocery and fast food products. Federal law does not require labeling of genetically engineered produce; however more than 20 states have introduced GMO labeling legislation.

The high consumption of these foods in the American diet has led to a surge in medical conditions that did not exist before the introduction of the product such as high inflammation, obesity, spontaneous abortions, birth defects, fertility issues in men and women to name a few. I have had to eliminate these foods from my diet completely due to the effects it has had on me. Look for items that are certified organic or bear the Non-GMO Project Verified Label. Organic certified products are not allowed to use GMOs. Just say No to GMO.

More important pieces of information that we all need to know about our food is whether our food is Hybrid, Acidic or Alkaline.

Hybrid:

Hybrid foods are foods which will not grow in nature. They are created when plant breeders intentionally cross-pollinate two different varieties of a plant, aiming to produce an offspring, or hybrid, that contains the best traits of each of the parents. One noteworthy feature of hybrid foods is that their seeds cannot germinate on their own. They require human intervention to grow. Cross-pollination, on the other hand, is a natural process that occurs within members of the same plant species.

The purpose of hybrid foods, when they were produced for the first time in the 1930s, was to help farmers produce crops on farms on which natural foods could not grow. As in much of the 19th century, the name of the game in the first few decades of the 20th century was mono-cropping. Every farmer, big or small, produced a single crop year after year. The result of years of mono-cropping was devastating. Aggressive mono-cropping, coupled with heavy, incessant use of pesticides and herbicides lead to large scale plant disease and made the soil unconducive. The solution, farmers, scientists, and governments agreed, was to produce hybrid foods.

Why aren't hybrid foods as healthy as natural foods? Unlike non-hybrid foods, hybrid foods have the following shortcomings: they have high sugar and starch content; In addition, the sugar present in hybrid foods is not completely absorbed or used by the pancreas and liver; they don't have proper mineral balance; Consumption of hybrid foods, over time, may lead to mineral imbalance; Some hybrid foods can worsen certain fungal conditions like Candida.

Some common hybrid fruits are: seedless apples, seedless citrus fruit, seedless grapes, and seedless watermelons. Common hybrid vegetables include beets, carrots, yellow corn, and white potatoes. Common hybrid nuts, seeds and beans include: cashews, oats, rice, wheat, wheat grass, soy, legumes, and most beans. Common hybrid herbs include: Goldenseal, Ginseng, Echinacea, Chamomile, Aloe Vera, Nutmeg, and Garlic. If you are fighting a chronic disease, eliminate these items from your diet. If you are trying to stay healthy, eat only occasionally.

Alkaline vs Acidic:

A 2012 review published in the Journal of Environmental Health found that balancing your body's pH through an alkaline diet can be helpful in reducing morbidity and mortality from numerous chronic diseases and ailments — such as hypertension, diabetes, arthritis, vitamin D deficiency, and low bone density, just to name a few.

Research shows that diets consisting of highly alkaline foods result in a more alkaline urine pH level, which helps protect healthy cells and balance essential mineral levels.

What we call pH is short for the potential of hydrogen. It's a measure of the acidity or alkalinity of our body's fluids and tissues. It's measured on a scale from 0 to 14. The more acidic a solution is, the lower its pH. The more alkaline, the higher the number is. A pH of around 7 is considered neutral, but since the optimal human body tends to be around 7.4, we consider the healthiest pH to be one that's slightly alkaline.

Whenever possible, try to buy organic alkaline foods. Experts feel that one important consideration in regard to eating an alkaline diet is to become knowledgeable about what type of soil your produce was grown in — since fruits and vegetables that are grown in organic, mineral-dense soil tend to be more alkalizing. Research shows that the type of soil that plants are grown in can significantly influence their vitamin and mineral content.

The ideal pH of soil for the best overall availability of essential nutrients in plants is between 6 and 7. Acidic soils below a pH of 6 may have reduced calcium and magnesium, and soil above a pH of 7 may result in chemically unavailable iron, manganese, copper and zinc. Soil that's well-rotated organically sustained and exposed to wildlife/grazing cattle tends to be the healthiest.

If you're curious to know your pH level before implementing these tips, you can test your pH by purchasing strips at your local health food store or pharmacy. You can measure your pH with saliva or urine. Your second urination of the morning will give you the best results. Compare the colors on your test strip to a chart that comes with your test strip kit. During the day, the best time to test your pH is one hour before a meal and two hours after a meal. If you test with your saliva, you want to try to stay between 6.8 and 7.2.

Anti-Alkaline Foods and Habits:

Foods that contribute most to acidity include:

- High-sodium foods: **Processed foods** contain tons of sodium chloride — table salt — which constricts blood vessels and creates acidity
- Cold cuts and conventional meats with nitrates

- Processed cereals (such as corn flakes)

- Eggs

- **Green** Lentils

- Peanuts

- Caffeinated drinks and alcohol

- Oats and whole wheat products: All grains, whole or not, create acidity in the body. Americans ingest most of their plant food quota in the form of processed corn or wheat.

- Milk: Calcium-rich dairy products cause some of the highest rates of osteoporosis. That's because they create acidity in the body! When your bloodstream becomes too acidic, it will steal calcium (a more alkaline substance) from the bones to try to balance out the pH level. So, the best way to **prevent** **osteoporosis** is to eat lots of alkaline green leafy veggies!

- Wheat pasta, rice, bread and packaged grain products

What other kinds of habits can cause acidity in your body? The biggest offenders include:

- Alcohol and drug use

- High caffeine intake

- Antibiotic overuse

- Artificial sweeteners

- Chronic stress

- Declining nutrient levels in foods due to industrial - farming

- Low levels of fiber in the diet

- Lack of exercise

- Over-exercise

- Excess animal meats in the diet (from non-grass-fed sources)

- Excess hormones from foods, health and beauty products and plastics

- Exposure to chemicals and radiation from household cleansers, building materials, computers, cell phones and microwaves

- Food coloring and preservatives

- Pesticides and herbicides

- Pollution

- Poor chewing and eating habits

- Processed and refined foods

- Shallow breathing

Other areas of concern on the food we intake are discussed below.

Sugar:

Today, an average American consumes about 32 teaspoons of sugar per day. New numbers came out in February 2015. The Washington Post did a story on it using grams (4 grams = 1 tsp). They quoted Euromonitor's study, which said Americans are now consuming 126 grams, which would equal close to 32 teaspoons. The amount of sugar adults consume each day is about 22 teaspoons a day. What's even more disturbing is that people are consuming excessive sugar in the form of fructose or high-fructose corn syrup (HFCS). This highly processed form of sugar is cheaper yet 20 percent sweeter than regular table sugar, which is why many food and beverage manufacturers decided to use it for their products, as it would allow them to save money in the long run.

It is unsurprising that an average American now consumes roughly 47 pounds of cane sugar and 35 pounds of high-fructose corn syrup every year. Artificial sweeteners aren't any better; they will cause you to crave even more sugar. According to the American Diabetic and Diabetic Association, increased sugar consumption is the leading cause of degenerative disease. It leads to many chronic illnesses such as acid reflux, migraines, joint pain, irritable bowel, anxiety, stress and fatigue. Fructose is linked to Insulin resistance and obesity, elevated blood pressure, elevated triglycerides and LDL (bad) cholesterol, depletion of vitamins and minerals, cardiovascular disease, liver disease, cancer, arthritis, and gout.

How to break the sugar addition:

- Make the decision to cut the sugar. Commit to 10 days without sugary foods.

- Quit all forms of sugar: white flour, artificial sweeteners, hydrogenated fats, MSG, and pre-packaged foods.

- Stop drinking sugary drinks: sodas, diet sodas and juices. Only drink water with lemon, lime, mint, cucumbers or some other fruit infusion.

- Add protein to every meal: eggs, nuts, seeds, fish, chicken, grass-fed meat.

- Eat non-starchy vegetables: zucchini, onions, peppers, brussel sprouts, broccoli, leafy greens, etc.

- Eat good fats with each meal: avocado, nuts, seeds, fish, coconut oil.

- Manage your stress: Cortisol raises with stresses which can cause sugar cravings.

- Quit gluten and dairy: You will have more energy and less chest congestion.

- Sleep: We need at least 8 hours of sleep. Improper sleep can drive you to eat.

Breaking the sugar addiction will help you break the sugar cravings. Limit sugar intake moving forward. Look for foods with a sugar content in the single digits on the label.

Soy based products:

For centuries, Asian people have been consuming fermented soy products such as natto, tempeh, and soy sauce, and enjoying the health benefits. Fermented soy does not wreak havoc on your body like unfermented soy products do. Ninety one percent of the soy grown in the United States is genetically engineered to impart resistance to the toxic herbicide Roundup, with which it's heavily sprayed. Unlike the Asian culture, where people eat small amounts of whole non-GMO soybean products, western food processors separate the soybean into two commodities—protein and oil. And there is nothing natural or safe about these products.

Unfortunately, many Americans who are committed to healthy lifestyles have been manipulated into believing that unfermented and processed soy products like tofu, soymilk, soy cheese, soy burgers and soy ice cream are good for them. From 1992 to 2006, soy food sales increased from $300 million to nearly $4 billion, practically overnight, according to the Soyfoods Association of North America. Soy has been added to almost all processed foods in the grocery store. As a test, go to the salad dressing section of your local grocery store and look at the ingredients. Almost all of them have soybean oil or soy lecithin as an ingredient even the ones that are supposed to have olive oil as the main ingredient.

Dr. Kaayla Daniel, author of The Whole Soy Story, points out thousands of studies linking soy to malnutrition, digestive distress, immune-system breakdown, thyroid dysfunction, dementia, hormonal imbalances, reproductive disorders, infertility, infant abnormalities, breast cancer, heart disease and an increase in allergies.

Soy is loaded with the isoflavones which is a type of phytoestrogen, which is a plant compound resembling human estrogen. These compounds mimic and sometimes block the hormone estrogen and have been found to have adverse effects on various human tissues. Soy phytoestrogens are known to disrupt endocrine function, may cause infertility, and may promote breast cancer in women. Drinking even two glasses of soymilk daily for one month provides enough of these compounds to alter a woman's menstrual cycle.

Nearly 20 percent of U.S. infants are now fed soy formula, but the estrogens in soy can irreversibly harm your baby's sexual development and reproductive health. When infants are fed soy formula, they take in an estimated five birth control pills' worth of estrogen every day and have up to 20,000 times the amount of estrogen in circulation as those fed other formulas! Problems may be demonstrated with the early onset of menstrual cycles in young girls.

Tips for Avoiding Unwanted Soy Foods:
For a simple rule of thumb, just remember that unless soy is fermented (tempeh, miso, natto, or traditionally made soy sauce), you're better off avoiding it.

Soy foods to avoid include: Tofu, TVP (texturized vegetable protein) or soy protein isolate, which contains a large amount of MSG, which you should definitely not consume, soybean oil, soymilk, soy cheese, soy ice cream, soy yogurt, Soy "meat" (meatless products made of TVP), soy protein, edamame and soy infant formula.

One other common source of soy is lecithin which is used as an emulsifier in many foods and supplements. These should be avoided as well.

The best way to eliminate non-fermented soy from your diet is to avoid all processed and fast foods and instead purchase whole foods that you prepare yourself. If you do buy packaged foods, you can check the label to see if it contains soy. The Food Allergen Labeling and Consumer Protection Act, which took effect in January 2006, requires that food manufacturers list soy on the label, because it's one of the top eight food allergens. So, even if soy is hidden in colors, flavors, or spice blends added to foods, it must be clearly stated on the label. I reiterate, read all food labels. Know what you are eating.

Meat:

I am vegan. I have found that it was best for me in my fight against fibroids. I ate grass-fed beef thinking that it would be okay. But eventually, that led me to excessive bleeding and a trip to the hospital. For me, it is best that I do not eat meat in this season in my life. Animals have hormones so if you eat meat; you are also ingesting their hormones.

If you choose to eat meat, choose healthy meats such as wild Alaskan or Pacific fish (Salmon, Mahi Mahi, Mackerel, or Halibut). Avoid Farmed-raised fish such as Tilapia. Select organic chicken or turkey, grass-fed beef or lamb. Eliminate Pork and Shellfish from your diet. These animals consume waste and excrement and their systems do not have a sophisticated method of filtering out toxins.

Pork consumption has been associated with diseases like liver cirrhosis, liver cancer, and multiple sclerosis (MS). Another problem with pork consumption is that Americans usually eat processed pork, which is preserved by smoking, curing or salting, or adding potentially harmful chemical preservatives such as nitrate which are clearly associated with an increased risk of certain cancers.

How to eliminate Estrogen Overload
- Eliminate Soy from your food and body products
- Eliminate Meat
- Eliminate Non-GMOs and Hybrid foods from your diet
- Transition to Natural Body Products
- Transition to Natural Household Cleaners and products
- Detox the Liver
- Build up your Immune System

THE TRANSITION PLAN

CHANGE, although it can be positive, it can sometimes be overwhelming. Thinking about all the things that need to be done or taken care of can be mentally exhausting. Therefore, taking one step at a time will help to ease the mental anguish. Remember, you can't do it all today.

When starting to transition to an organic and natural lifestyle, you should begin with simple things that you can change. Then add new changes a little at a time. For example, if you're use to eating a lot of carbs, cut the amount in half. If you're used to eating bread at every meal, eat bread at only one meal. Not a person who exercises? Start taking a 5 minute walk a day and add 5 minutes each month until you can walk 20 minutes to an hour a day or at least 3-4 times a week. Need help drinking water? Try adding lemon, lime or cucumber to help add taste. There is always something you can do better than what you are doing. If your body is not use to even the smallest change, making that small change is going to alert your body that something is different, and you should see or feel a difference.

Make a commitment to yourself to improve your health. Create a plan in writing on how you are going to make healthy changes. Enter dates and times for exercise on your weekly planner.

Food:

Eat fresh, organic, non-GMO, non-hybrid foods. Soak all fruits and vegetables in equal parts vinegar and water. Peel all fruits and vegetables. Buy food in glass jars, waxed cardboard or tin cans marked with 'no BPA lining' on the labels. Don't buy foods in plastic containers marked "pc" or "recycling #7".

Buying organic or from local food sources will help you to avoid toxic pesticides used on conventional produce. See ewg.org for the full list of foods with the highest concentration of pesticides. Number 1 and 2 are spinach and strawberries.

Cooking Food:

Food should only be cooked by simmering, steaming, baking or roasting. Food is best eaten raw or cooked at a medium high temperature. Food should never be fried.

Prepared Foods:

When you purchase pre-packaged food, look for foods that contain organic, non-GMO and non-hybrid ingredients. As more and more people are making healthier choices for their food supplies, companies are making foods to cash in on this consumer base. I am surprised and amazed at the volume of choices there are to choose from that fits my dietary lifestyle.

Always, always read the labels of pre-packaged food to ensure you are not ingesting anything that may harm you, especially soy. Because many vegans do not eat meat but do eat soy, a lot of prepared foods contain this ingredient. Do not purchase it if it contains soy.

Meal Plans:

Phase out microwave meals. Most are high in salt or sugar and/or contain preservatives or items you don't want to consume.

Create a meal plan for the week.

Commit to cooking more home cooked meals. Start with making one meal in the week and add an additional meal every week.

Most people eat the same five or six meals each week. Become familiar with easy meals and add to it every week. As you become more familiar, it won't take as long to make each meal.

When writing the grocery list, list the foods in the order they are located in the grocery store. You won't need to waste time walking back and forth across the store.

Processed foods are located on the inside aisles. Aim for more fresh foods. The bulk of your groceries should be found on the outside aisles in the fruits, vegetables, fresh meats, non-dairy sections.

Practice meal prepping. Pick a day of the week to grocery shop. Soak fruits and vegetables in vinegar and water for five minutes, rinse and pat dry.

Purchase wire racks to hold your fresh fruits and vegetables on the counter. This will keep them in front of you. The goal is to eat them up before the next week's grocery run. If they start ripening too fast, place them in the refrigerator to halt the ripening process.

Pick another day to chop/cut/slice vegetables for recipes. You can store all vegetables for one meal together and pre-mix spices or sauces. When dinner time comes, all you will need to do is dump it in the pot or pan and simmer.

There are several companies that provide meals online. Each meal comes with the ingredients and the instructions on how to make the meal. They also cater to specialized diets.

You can find thousands of recipes suited for your tastes on the app, Pinterest or on You Tube. You can search on words or phrases like 'meal prep', 'vegetarian meals', 'soups', 'salads' or search for one ingredient you would like to use such as 'coconut flour'.

You can also load apps on your phone or iPad as well as download eBooks from kindle or other sources. Watch a cooking network to get inspired. I watch the cooking show 'Chopped' on the Food Network as I prepare dinner. It makes it more fun and less of a chore. This is a good time to get your children involved in making healthy meals.

Eating Out:
Review the menu before you go to the restaurant. Many restaurants post theirs online. Decide what to order before you get to the restaurant.

Eliminate sugary sodas and juices. Make a habit of asking for water, water with lemon or hot water with lemon. You may also request an unsweet tea or hot tea. Carry packets of stevia with you and use as your sweetener. Eventually, this will become a habit and you will save a couple of bucks on the meal.

Skip the bread or hors d'oeuvres. Select salads, vegetable soups (non-creamy), cold water fish (salmon, mahi-mahi, mackerel, halibut) from the Alaskan or Pacific oceans, grass fed beef /lamb, chicken/turkey (preferably organic), healthy grains or starches. Many restaurants serve steamed vegetables, quinoa and butternut squash.

Phase out Fast Food and opt for Fast Casual:
As you commit to preparing your weekly meals, it will become easier to eliminate eating at fast food restaurants. Eventually, all of your meals and snacks will already be available.

Occasionally, you may not want to eat at home or spend the money to eat at a fancy restaurant. To fill in the gap, select a fast-casual restaurant.

A fast-casual restaurant is a type of restaurant that does not offer full table service but promises a higher quality of food with fewer frozen or processed ingredients than a fast food restaurant. A few restaurants that fall in this category are Jason's Deli, Panera Bread, Chipotle Mexican Grill and Zoe's Kitchen to name a few. The list of restaurants in this genre is growing longer each year.

Also look for restaurants in your area that serve Farm to Table meals. Some of them have gardens on site or purchase their ingredients from local farmers.

GROCERIES

Transition to organic produce. Although some of these foods may be more expensive, think of it as an investment in yourself. Major grocery store chains are carrying a large selection of organic produce along with foods without GMOS and preservatives. The prices are decreasing as consumers are demanding natural foods. For example, the grocery store, Harris Teeter, now carries foods with the label "Free From 101" indicating these items are free from 101 artificial preservatives and ingredients. Other grocers such as Kroger's and Aldi's also offer a wide range of organic foods at reasonable prices.

I'm blessed to have two natural food co-ops, two major natural food store chains, a country store and several farmer's markets in my home town. Look for local cooperative stores in your area. When you join a co-op, you are a co-owner in the store. A few months ago, I joined my local co-op for a $25 annual fee where I receive

10% off all of my purchases. The store cashier compared the $25 annual fee to purchasing a membership at a bulk store. The prices of the food items at the co-op are comparable and many times much less than the major food chains. If you would like to locate a co-op near you, check out the Independent Natural Food Retailers Association for a list of stores in your area: naturalfoodretailers.net/member-directory.

Let's Begin:

I know I have covered a lot of information about food and its importance to your healing. By changing the foods, I ate on a daily basis, I was able to decrease the estrogen, lose weight and had shorter and lighter menstrual cycles.

The foods on the lists below have been adapted from two sources, Dr. Sebi's theory on eliminating disease and the book, Got fibroids? ® The Fibroid Elimination Bible by Dr. Amsu Anpu & Dr. Amun Neb.

FOOD SUBSTITUTIONS

Promotes Poor Health	*Promotes Healing*
White / Brown Rice Couscous	Quinoa, Spelt, Wild Rice Black Rice aka. Forbidden Rice
Oatmeal, Grits Cream of Wheat	Millet, Amaranth, Teff, Quinoa or Quinoa Flakes
White / Sweet Potatoes Turnips, Rutabagas	Wild Yams, Purple Potatoes, Butternut Squash Acorn Squash
Kidney beans, Black-eyed peas White beans, Baked beans Green lentils	Black/Navy/Adzuki beans Garbanzo/Chickpeas Red lentils Green-snap beans
Wheat Bread (gluten)	Spelt, Sprouted, Sourdough Rye bread (without soy)
White Flour	Spelt/Almond/Coconut flour Garbanzo/Chickpea flour Teff flour
White Cane Sugar	Date Sugar, Coconut Sugar Raw Honey, Maple Syrup *(Limit these sugars to 1 TBSP/day)*
Splenda (sucralose), Equal and NutraSweet (aspartame) Sweet/N Low (saccharin)	Stevia, Xylitol

Corn Starch	Arrowroot Starch
Wheat pasta / macaroni / spaghetti	Spelt, Chickpea, Lentil, Black bean pasta / macaroni / spaghetti
Wheat or Rice Asian Noodles	Kelp or Miracle Noodles (zero Calories ~ found in the Asian Foods section)
White Onions	Red Onions, Scallions
Green Bell Peppers	Sweet Bell Peppers
Peanuts / Peanut Butter	Raw - Almonds, Walnuts, Brazil nuts / Almond Butter
Seeds	Raw - Pumpkin, Hemp, Chia, Black Sesame seeds
Spinach	Callaloo, Swiss Chard, Kale
Garlic	Horseradish, Chives
Dairy Milk	Almond, Coconut, Hemp Milk
Margarine, Butter	Coconut Butter
Canola, Corn, Sunflower, Safflower, Vegetable oil	Olive, Coconut, Almond, Avocado, Sesame Oil
Mayo	Hummus, Avocado, Pesto
Soy Sauce	Coconut Amino Sauce

Yellow Corn	Blue Corn
Yellow Corn Chips	Blue Corn Chips
	Purple Potato Chips
Yellow Corn Tortillas	Spelt Tortillas
Table Salt	Pink Himalayan,
	Black Hawaiian
	Celtic Sea Salt

* Add Sea Kelp or Dulce / Nori, Wakame, Arame Seaweed to your diet to replace the iodine you were getting from table salt

TIP

It is less expensive to purchase grains, nuts and seeds from the bulk bins than buying them individually wrapped.

For example, Quinoa purchased from the bulk bin is priced at $2.99 lb. Quinoa purchased in a pre-packaged bag costs $4.99 per 12 oz. or $6.65 lb. Buying in bulk will save you $3.66 per lb.

Foods That Promote Healing

Fruit

Apples (green/red), All berries except cranberries, Avocados, Pears (green/purple), Grapefruit (seeded), Grapes (purple seeded), Jackfruit, Lemons, Limes, Key Limes, Mangoes (red), Mangosteen, Seeded Melons (Cantaloupe, Honey Dew, Watermelon), Pineapples, Pitted Fruit (Nectarines, Peaches, Plums), Prickly Pear (Cactus Fruit), Plantains, Soursops

Vegetables

Artichokes, Broccoli, Brussel Sprouts, Callaloo (Amaranth greens), Cauliflower, Choyote (Mexican) Squash, Izote – Cactus Flower/Cactus Leaf, Cucumber, Celery, Fenugreek, Horseradish, Kale, Nopales (Mexican Cactus), Olives, Yellow/Zucchini Squash, Grape/Roma Tomatoes, Okra, Collard Greens, Dandelion Greens, Mustard Greens, Poke Salad (Greens), Green/Red Cabbage, Arugula, Romaine Lettuce, Tomatillo, Watercress, Sea Vegetables (Dulse/Arame/Hijiki/Nori), Kelp, Purple Moss

Herbs and Spices

Basil, Bay Leaf, Cayenne, Chives, Cinnamon, Cumin, Curry, Dill, Oregano, Smoked Paprika, Tarragon

It's also less expensive to purchase food in season
rather out of season.

Spring   *Mid-March to Mid-June*

Apricots, artichokes, avocados, berries, cherries, grapefruit, lemons, lettuce, melons, peaches, plums, strawberries, wild greens

Summer   *Mid-June to Mid-September*

Apples, avocados, basil, bell peppers, berries, cherries, cilantro, cucumbers, figs, grapes, mangoes, nectarines, peaches, peppers, summer squash, tomatoes, watermelon, zucchini

Autumn   *Mid-September to Mid-December*

Arugula, broccoli, brussel sprouts, coconut, collards, fennel, grapes, kale, limes, pears, shallots, swiss chard, winter squash

Winter   *Mid-December to Mid-March*

Cabbage, celery, citrus, dates, onions, pears, pineapple

RECIPES

Fruit Bowl Serving: 1

2 cups fruit, sliced
1 tablespoon hemp or chia seeds or both
¼ cup walnuts
¼ cup unsweetened shredded coconut (optional)
½ cup non-dairy milk (optional)
Fruit can be any combination of fruit you have on hand.
Sprinkle fruit with seeds, nuts and coconut. Pour milk
over the mixture and eat like cereal.

Millet   Serving: 1

½ cup millet
1 cup water
1 tablespoon coconut oil
½ teaspoon sea salt
1 teaspoon cinnamon
1 teaspoon sweetener of your choice
1 cup non-dairy milk
3 dates chopped (optional)
¼ cup chopped nuts (optional)

Simmer the millet in the water at medium high heat for
20 minutes. Remove from the eye and let sit for 10
minutes. Add the remaining ingredients.

Follow this recipe for Teff and Amaranth by following the instructions on the package for correct water measurements.

Pancakes   Servings: 2

1 cup spelt flour
2 tablespoons coconut sugar
2 ½ teaspoons baking powder
½ teaspoon salt
1 egg substitute (or 1 egg)
1 teaspoon vanilla flavoring
3 tablespoons melted coconut oil
1 ¼ cup non-dairy milk
Maple syrup

Mix dry. Mix wet. Beat dry and wet together. Heat skillet on medium heat. Melt a teaspoon on coconut oil in the pan. Scoop ¼ cup batter in the hot pan. Flip pancake when bubbles from on top. Serve with maple syrup.

Chickpea Salad   Servings: 4

1 12 oz. can or 1½ cups cooked chickpeas, drained
1 avocado
1 tablespoon lemon juice
1 teaspoon turmeric
4 chopped Kalamata olives
Salt and pepper to taste

Mash chickpeas and avocado. Leave some lumps. Fold in other ingredients.

Serve on toasted bread with lettuce, sliced tomato, red onions.

Spicy Beans   Servings: 4

1 12 ounce can or 1½ cups cooked Black beans
1 12 ounce can diced tomatoes with green chilies
½ red onion chopped
1 tablespoon coconut oil
1 tablespoon chili powder
1 teaspoon cayenne pepper, cumin, cinnamon

Turn skillet on medium heat. Sauté onions for 5 minutes. Add remaining ingredients and simmer 15-20 minutes.

Grillable Black Bean Burger Servings: 6

3 cups rinsed black beans
1 egg substitute (or 1 egg)
½ cup gluten free bread crumbs
½ cup butternut squash puree
½ teaspoon salt
¼ teaspoon cumin, oregano, garlic powder, turmeric

In the food processor, pulse 2 cups of black beans, bread crumbs, squash until chunky. Add egg and spices.

Transfer to a bowl and add remaining cup of beans. Mix with hands and form burgers. Cook on medium low heat. Serve on gluten free buns with toppings.

Oven Steamed Brussel Sprouts   Servings: 2

½ pound Brussel sprouts, ends cut off, sliced in half
1 lemon sliced
Salt and pepper to taste

Preheat oven on 400 degrees. Prepare baking dish by lining it with a large piece of foil. Place parchment paper on top of the foil. Pour the Brussel sprouts in the dish on top of the parchment paper. Sprinkle with salt and pepper. Place sliced lemons on top. Wrap the parchment paper and foil to seal the Brussel sprouts. Bake in the oven for 40 minutes or until tender.

Roasted Butternut Squash   Servings: 4

4 cups raw, cubed butternut squash
2 tablespoon melted coconut oil
3 tablespoon maple syrup
1 teaspoon cinnamon
2 cups chopped walnuts
1 cup dried tart cherries

Preheat oven to 400 degrees. Toss squash with oil, syrup, and cinnamon. Place in baking dish into the oven. Roast

30 minutes or until tender. Remove from oven and add walnuts and cherries.

Black Bean Salad   Servings: 4

1 12 oz. can or 1½ cups cooked black beans, rinsed
1 cup cherry tomatoes, sliced in half
½ cup chopped red onions
2 tablespoons olive oil
½ lime juice

Mix all together.

Double Chocolate Pudding Pots   Servings: 4

1 large ripe plantain
2 avocados
¼ cup cacao powder
½ cup + 2 Tablespoons maple syrup
3 tablespoons Enjoy Life chocolate chips, melted
1 box Enjoy Life Brownie Cookies
Fresh berries for garnish

In a high-speed blender, puree plantain, avocados, cacao powder, and maple syrup while adding milk 1 Tablespoon at a time until smooth. Crumble 1 cookie in a dish. Spoon pudding on top. Add another crumbled cookie and pudding. Top with berries. Repeat with other cups and serve.

RESOURCES

<u>Books</u>

Got Fibroids The Fibroid Elimination Bible
by Dr. Amsu Anpu & Dr. Amun Neb

Forks Over Knives: The Plant-Based Way to Health
By Gene Stone and T. Colin Campbell

Maximized Living Nutrition Plans
by Dr. B.J. Hardick, Kimberly Roberto
and Dr. Ben Lerner

<u>YouTube</u>

Dr. Eric Berg
Dr. Josh Axe
Gessie Thompson
Dr. Sebi: Eat to Live

<u>Documentaries</u>

Forks Over Knives
Sugar Coated
Cowspiracy: The Sustainability Secret
Fat, Sick, & Nearly Dead
Food Matters
Fed Up
Super Size Me
Vegucated

Websites

Mercola.com
Draxe.com
Ewg.org
Fibroidelimination.com
Hopebeyondfibroids.com
Forksoverknives.com
Energyfanatics,com
Purityfoods.com
alkalinegourmet.net
Thrivemarket.com
Amazon.com
Bobsredmill.com
Vitacost.com
Swansonvitamins.com
Vitaminshoppe.com
Activeherbs.com
Renuherbs.com

www.ingramcontent.com/pod-product-compliance
Lightning Source LLC
Chambersburg PA
CBHW022120280326
41933CB00007B/479